A 5-Prong Approach to Handling
Cancer Diagnosis & Treatment

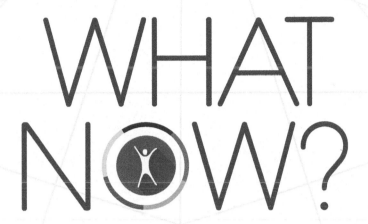

WHAT
NOW?

R. CRAIG COPPOLA

What Now? A 5-Prong Approach to Handling Cancer Diagnosis & Treatment

Habanero Publishing, LLC
6040 E. Montecito Ave
Scottsdale, AZ 85251

Copyright © 2018, R. Craig Coppola

Published in the United States of America

ISBN-13: 978-0-9898672-9-0

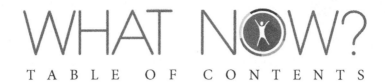

WHAT NOW?

TABLE OF CONTENTS

Introduction

Sit at a computer and Google "Getting through cancer." What comes up? Lots of motivational books on survival after cancer, but very few about what to do immediately after your first diagnosis and throughout treatment.

When I was diagnosed and went looking for guidance, I didn't find much practical and to-the-point help for each phase of my treatment. I was stuck after my initial diagnosis, asking myself the same question you are: "What now?"

Throughout my cancer diagnosis and treatment, I felt like there were so many things that were left unsaid and undocumented. I learned very quickly during the process that cancer is a business for the hospitals and doctors, and while they may care deeply about their patients, no one cares more about your health than you do.

I read a book once by a man who had been diagnosed with prostate cancer. The title was, *There Is No They, There's Only You.* The book was about how people always ask, "What do *they* say?" What do the doctors, the specialists, the oncologists, say?

I'm here to tell you that there is no "they." So stop asking what they say and start asking yourself, "What do *I* want? And what do *I* want to do?"

From the very first moment you receive your first diagnosis until the end of treatment, if you're not controlling your own process and thinking about what you want and what you're going to do, then you're at the mercy of the system. If you are like me, that doesn't cut it. You want to control your own destiny.

Everyone reading this will have a unique situation and will approach each phase of their treatment and process differently. This is exactly what I advocate. There is no one-size-fits-all for cancer treatment. You have to do what feels right to you in your personal situation.

I wrote this guide to offer my own process and how I dealt with every phase of my treatment, not so that you can follow it exactly, but so that you can refer to it and make your own plan. It doesn't matter what your diagnosis is, what your financial situation is, or what your goals are. The most important thing is that you have a plan that works for you.

The 5-Prong Approach

Upon receiving the news that I had lymphoma, I sat down and thought about how I would fight it. I came up with a four-prong approach, and then added a fifth prong after treatments began.

The original four prongs were:

1. **Medical Care**—I wanted to get to the best doctors in the world. I wanted to get multiple opinions and come up with a treatment plan that I felt confident in as quickly as possible.

2. **Holistic Approach**—I wanted to do what I could for myself during this process beyond the medical treatment. I wanted to approach it from a holistic mindset, addressing all aspects of my life together.

3. **Spiritual Considerations**—I wanted to explore my Christian faith and other faiths in deeper ways. I wanted to be open and accepting of all I could ingest.

4. **Setting Goals**—I set up goals for myself, inside and outside of my health goals. I wanted to look back at the time spent fighting cancer and say it was worth it—whether I went into remission or not—and that I got some things done that were on my goals list anyway. These included some big goals (get my book published) and some small ones (hike daily).

5. **Expect the Unexpected**—After treatments began, I started experiencing things I was not prepared

for in a number of different ways. Looking back, that should not have been surprising. Keep in mind, I set my system up when I was healthy. I was asymptomatic at the time of diagnosis, so I believed I could do most anything. When that didn't occur, I had to readjust.

Throughout all of the chemo and radiation, I discovered that I didn't always have the ability to meet the above goals. That is when I added the fifth prong: expect the unexpected. When things came up, I thought about the issues, made decisions, and moved on.

It's important to remember that your plan is going to change. You have to be flexible to the unexpected happening. At each curve in the road, be prepared to refocus your plan and keep what's working for you.

In looking back, especially now that I'm cancer-free, I am 100% sure that I handled the process the right way for me.

I hope this book inspires you to stand strong, do what you want to do, and take your own path, not anyone else's.

To Your Health!

Craig

Throughout this book, I have included excerpts from my Caring Bridge site (www.caringbridge.org) of my personal journey to fight and beat cancer. I will explain more about this site later in the book.

My Story

On Monday, July 15, 2013, I woke up with a bump on the side of my neck. It was roughly the size of a golf ball and definitely had not been there the night before. By 10:45 that morning, I was getting it looked at by my general doctor. He felt I should get a scan, which I arranged to have at noon. The next day I had a meeting with a doctor at 11:45 who told me that the CT scan showed abnormally large lymph nodes. He said I should schedule a biopsy. Five days before the bump on my neck I was reading in bed and felt a hard-like muscle on my abs. I had the CT scan nurse scan that area also. Guess what—the scan showed very large lymphs in the abdomen as well.

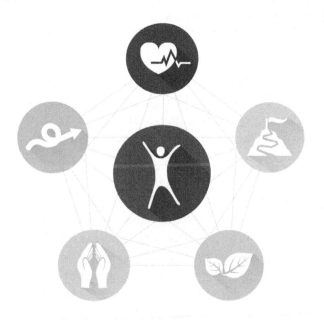

PRONG 1
MEDICAL CARE

Quarterback Your Care
at All Levels

There are a lot of cooks, and only one chef.
~ R. Craig Coppola

When you or someone you love receive the unimaginable news that you have cancer, you will face a lot of emotions and reactions. Unfortunately, there are also a lot of decisions you need to make, some of them right away.

Putting aside the emotions and focusing on the practical is extremely difficult. Right about now you're probably wondering how you're going to do that. How do you move past the shock of this news and get started?

Make YOUR Plan

Your first order of business is to create a plan. In the coming weeks, you will receive a lot of questions and opinions from doctors, friends, family, and acquaintances. At times, it will be very overwhelming, which is why I can't stress enough that you *MUST* create and implement your own plan. Cancer is not one of those things in life you can wing at the last minute. You have to get your arms around the situation fast. Remember, you are the quarterback of your health and your treatment. It's up to you to call the shots.

There will be multiple facets of your plan. I've included my 5 prongs in this book, but maybe you have more or less. What's important is that your plan includes the areas that are vital to you and you alone. No one can create your plan for you, not even your doctors.

When I received the news that I had lymphoma, my first step was to get the proper diagnosis and create a treatment strategy. Having this plan of action in place from the very beginning was extremely helpful. When people asked me questions or gave suggestions, it was far easier to thank them for their concern but stick to the process that worked best for me.

If you aren't sure where to start with your plan, begin by clarifying your priorities. What are the most important things to you? What things do you want to make sure come first in the next few weeks?

At the very top of the list should be your health. Before anything else, you have to get a handle on your diagnosis and treatment. That's where the medical care prong of your plan comes in.

Diagnosis

The first step in your plan is to get the right diagnosis. You want to know your diagnosis down to the smallest details. The best way to do that is to set up meetings with multiple doctors to get multiple opinions.

I am sure that you will receive many doctor referrals from family and friends. Take these referrals and start making appointments. No matter how confident a doctor seems, you *MUST* get more than one opinion on your diagnosis and care.

I was fortunate enough to travel around the country to meet with those who I thought were the best doctors for my type of cancer. This may not be possible for everyone, but you can and absolutely must get more than one opinion, no matter where the doctors are located. At a minimum, find the best three doctors for your specific type of cancer, in the nearest city to you. Make sure they specialize in your type of cancer, and set up an appointment with them in person.

I'll stress that last part again: *Always meet with the doctors and staff face-to-face*. You have to look the doctor in the eye and ask the questions you need answered. Do not accept no for an answer when it comes to getting a doctor's appointment. Trust me, they will move their calendars around to get you in. Doctors do care.

Meeting Your Doctors

Once you have your appointments made, it's time to start doing your homework. Do a little background research on the doctor you're meeting. What's their specialty? Who recommends them? Where are they located?

You will also want to do some reading on your own cancer diagnosis. All this will help you be prepared for your appointments.

Your main goal in these meetings is to *get your diagnosis done properly*, to get a consensus on your treatment, and then to work the treatment.

Make this main goal your top priority—always. This is important in life, but especially in your situation. So keep your focus on this goal as you prepare for the appointments.

Write down your questions before you arrive and remember to take someone with you to ask the questions you will forget or don't realize you have. I cannot recommend having an advocate enough. This is a stressful and emotional time for you, meaning things will fall between the cracks. Having someone who can remain objective and organized is a great bonus.

During your appointments, ask probing questions. Re-ask your questions until you are satisfied with the answers. Remember, you only get one sit down with this doctor to go over your diagnosis and plan. So make sure you ask all your questions and get all your answers in the first go around.

It's important to remember as you meet with these doctors, that at the end of the day, it's your health, not theirs. Every doctor means well, so take all their advice and opinions into consideration. But make your own decisions about what is best for you. You control your health. You are your best advocate!

You might also want to consult specialists, so make sure you understand which doctors to see and set those appointments up too. Oncologists see chemo patients, stem cell doctors see transplant patients, radiologists oversee radiation treatments, and surgeons of all types see surgery patients. They all have voices to add, but they all have their biases too. You need to be sure that you understand those biases as you meet with them. Over time, you will know their strengths and be able to weigh their opinions based on their training and education.

If you don't know where to start preparing for a doctor's visit, check out the resources below:

The American Cancer Society has worksheets you can download and bring to your doctor's appointments. Visit their website and download some of their questionnaires: www.cancer.org

The National Cancer Institute also has its own list of questions you should ask at your appointments: www.cancer.gov

Making a Treatment Plan

After your meetings with doctors and specialists, you will have to make a decision on your treatment plan. Every doctor will have their own opinion on your treatment plan, and the best-case scenario is that they will all agree on the same course of treatment. That doesn't always happen, however, so make sure you ask probing questions about treatment in your meetings so that you can make an informed decision about which course of action is right for you.

One way to feel confident in your treatment plan is by conducting your own research. There are always new technologies and treatments that become available. Make sure to research all cutting-edge options and seek out trusted advisors to share their own thoughts and feedback.

I went to some key people that I know to help me in my research. Ray Kurzweil and Dr. Peter Diamandis are two leading tech experts and entrepreneurs who are plugged into the latest developments in many different innovative areas of research. I turned to their exploration of bioresearch to keep up to date on the latest advancements. Ray is the author of *Transcend: Nine Steps to Living Well Forever*, and he knows almost all of the cutting-edge procedures.

I met with TGEN, the Translational Genomics Research Institute, which is at the cutting edge of genetic research. I also worked with Dr. Eric Cobb, my partner in Z Health, who also remains informed about the latest treatments and exercises.

Finally, a lot of people I know kept their family doctor on their team – even as a quarterback – to help them sift through the biases and perspectives of different professionals. It's a great option if you aren't sure where to start or who to listen to.

There are numerous other resources out there that you can use to start educating yourself. It's important to have at minimum a basic knowledge of what's happening in modern research so that you can ask your doctor if any of those treatments are right for you. But you won't know to ask unless you do your homework first.

Be prepared for opinions from everyone. You will be bombarded by suggestions from not only doctors but other survivors, well-wishers, friends and family, etc. They all have something to share with you, from super foods to eat (like broccoli), holistic treatments (like acupuncture and Chinese herbs), and so many more.

Thank them for their suggestions, choose the ones that sound appealing to you, and discard the others. This is your life.

You can even find thousands of options on the Internet. Feel free to review and research what you want, but then make *YOUR* plan the priority.

Once you collect all the opinions and data, you're in a far better position to make an informed choice about your treatment. Here, it's important to remember again that hospitals are businesses and doctors make a living off cancer. Every doctor you meet is going to have an opinion on your treatment, and will try to sell you. Go with *YOUR* instinct. Stand firm on what feels right to you and meets your needs.

Location, Location, Location

Once you get a treatment plan in place, your next big decision is choosing where to get this treatment and the doctor that goes with it.

Getting the best treatment possible given your circumstances is paramount. This will be different for everyone, depending on your personal and financial situations.

Ideally, your treatment will occur somewhere close to home, but if not, have someone on your team help you make arrangements to travel and/or lodge somewhere close to your treatment center. Again, everyone's plan will look different, so tend to your needs first.

Get a Team You Trust

One of the most important steps in the early days of your diagnosis is to put together a team that will support you throughout your treatment.

Your team is vital to your treatment. These are the people who will help you execute your plan, who will take care of various tasks so that you can focus on the most important things. Therefore, not only do you need to trust the people on your team, but you must like them as well.

Your team will include doctors, nurses, and assistant nurses, but it will also include non-medical team members who have your best interest at heart.

The people on your team will help you with important items outside your health care that need to be addressed. Create a list of the top 10 or 20 things on your plate, and decide who will take care of each item. Then, quickly delegate those tasks. Make sure everyone you delegate to is someone you trust 100%.

For many people, their team will consist of family members. I was fortunate enough to have people and resources available to me. Others will have to go looking for this support system, but trust me, these people are out there and they do want to help.

Some examples of team members you need may be:

- Someone to deal with your health insurance, bills, etc. This is an important item on the list, as one of the biggest concerns with cancer is how to handle your diagnosis from a financial perspective. The sooner that you or someone you trust gets to your insurance and finds out the details, the more time you will have to focus on your plan.

- Someone to take care of filing for disability income.

- Someone to update your will.

- Someone to take over any of your business-related items.

- Someone to handle your finances.

- Someone to book travel plans (as well as housing if you are going out of your community).

The sooner these items are off your plate, the faster you can focus on your plan.

BEGINNING TREATMENT

Your plan is in place. You have your diagnosis, you've gotten multiple opinions, and chosen your treatment path. All that preparation comes to fruition as you start your treatment.

Like everything you've done so far, you must have a plan for how you will tackle treatment. You can't show up for your first day unprepared. You have to account for every detail, or you will be at the mercy of your doctors and medicine.

> Written July 28, 2013
>
> So.....I have a journey ahead. I am turning my businesses over to all of my wonderful team. Andrew Cheney will be running my brokerage business. Brad Lemon will be quarterbacking my other businesses as well as a home office for investments, etc. This whole experience is made so much easier because I have great advisers, friends, and consultants who I have worked with for decades.

Again, conducting research and asking the right questions will serve you well here. If you do your homework ahead of time, you'll have a better idea of how treatment will affect you, what the routine will look like, and how you can physically and mentally prepare yourself.

Hospital Routines

If your treatment plan involves chemo, or any extended time spent in a hospital, have a plan in place for how you will spend that time.

During my first hospital stay, I quickly fell into routine that worked for me. I made sure to customize my stay every time I checked in so that I had some control over my health and my life.

Here are some tips to help you make the most of your hospital stay.

Make your hospital stay as comfortable as possible. Set your room up the way you like it. Bring your favorite blanket or pillow from home. Drape blankets over the windows and the machines to make it dark and easier to sleep. These little touches of comfort make a big difference in your treatment.

I made three signs for every hospital stay:

- Patient name is Craig. (They kept calling me Richard.)
- Patient is resting, please do not disturb. See nurse if emergency.
- Internet login number on the back of the door.

Come Prepared Hospitals have everything you *need*, but not everything you *want*. Make sure to pack the things you'll want for your treatment. Here are some of the items I always made sure to bring with me:

- Six bottles of water.
- My own blankets (one for bed and one for couch) and UGG® slippers to be cozy.
- A towel, dumbbells, wristbands, and blue band for workouts.
- POWERADE® Zero or other drinks. (Water is awful during chemo.)
- Have Desitin® for rashes.
- Use natural soap. (Odors will make you nauseous.)

Be sure you know the protocol. Nurses are busy, and they don't always have time to stop and explain what they're doing. Every time they come in, ask why and what they are doing. You get all kinds of drugs, not just chemo. They must have a good explanation for you to take whatever it is that they bring you. Remember, *YOU* are in control of *YOUR* health.

During my stays, I said no to blood-thinning shots, and Monitor E Care (a 24-hour monitor that was intrusive). I knew I didn't want these things, but had to make that clear to the nurses every time I checked in.

Write down questions for doctors' visits. You usually only get one doctor's visit a day in the hospital, and sometimes not even that if you are in an outpatient clinic. So be prepared for every precious minute of your doctor's time that you can get. Have your questions and concerns written down ahead of time, so you don't miss anything.

Minimize interruptions. Nurses, doctors, and orderlies will be coming in and out at all hours of the day. Sometimes, you just want some peace and quiet. Minimize interruptions by telling the head nurse, "I am going to nap for 90 minutes now. Please, no interruptions." Maybe put a sign on the door that says, "Napping. Come back at 5:00."

I also maintained a very clear night schedule:

- All vitals and work should be done before 9 PM.
- There should be no interruptions until rounds at 5 AM or later.

Setting these expectations early helped me get plenty of rest, which was paramount for my health.

Find a way to make the stay a positive experience. Some suggestions are to work out every day. I hit the treadmill every day I was in the hospital, but you might want to add some stretching or a couple rounds of yoga. It is a great time to catch up on TV or reading. Find a television series *(Game of Thrones, Entourage, Scandal)* that you've wanted to binge watch, read a book or listen on tape, have cards and games for kids' visits, etc. There's a lot of down time during your hospital stay, so make sure you come prepared to fill those hours.

Do not eat lunch or dinner in the hospital cafeteria. Breakfast is good in the hospital—who can mess up eggs? But when it comes to other meals, get them from outside the hospital. Invite people to join you for meals. Your friends and family want to bring you food. Tell your friends and family what you want; they will bring it. They WANT to help.

I made a calendar and scheduled a dinner with a different friend for every night of my stay. Not only did they bring delicious meals, but they made me laugh and forget about my time in the hospital.

Non-Hospital Treatments

If your treatment plan doesn't include overnight or extended stays in the hospital, some of these suggestions still apply to you. Bring your comfy blanket to chemo sessions. Ask questions every time you go. Have friends or family keep you company. The more you can do to take ownership of your treatment, the less you will feel like a number.

Between Treatments

Once your treatment is finished and you return home, immediately take back your life. I went hiking as soon as I got home after my first session—at 4 AM. I drove home, put my shoes on, and hit the trail. Within an hour of my release, I had my life back. Then I took a nap.

After hospital stay two, my daughter taught me some moves that were part of "Shake it off," a volleyball saying—foot stomps, hands shaking in the air. Let it go ASAP.

Between chemo rounds you get a certain number of days to live your life, so live it. Limit business (or be in business the way you want to be involved), dedicate some time to catching up with your friends, nap, and work out on your schedule.

Don't make commitments. It's easier to say, "I might show up, but if I don't feel up to it, then I won't." This is better than saying, "I will be there" and not showing up due to complications.

What brings you joy? Where do you find peace? What refreshes you? Don't accept treatments as "lost" time. Find ways to keep your mind and body active, whenever possible.

What Happens Between Rounds of Chemo

Written August 16, 2013 1:02 p.m.

Friday 8/16/13. I have been out of the hospital for ten days and thought I would update you on what goes on during the two weeks between chemo sessions.

Before I update the last ten days, I am headed back in for round two on Monday (8/19). One of my big items was to make sure I was not "dreading" going back in for 120 hours of continuous chemo drip and isolation on the fifth floor of Banner Gateway Hospital. I think I am ready.

To get ready, here is a bit of my strategy:

*1—**Spend every day out of the hospital** on some aspect getting organized for round two.*

*2—**Set goals for my session**. Here are a few for round two: A—listen to at least 5 meditation tapes to see which ones work for me (I have acquired over 12), B-watch season two of Game of Thrones,*

C-Catch every sunrise on the treadmill, etc. There are more. I am not trying to change the world, just trying to feel like I accomplish something each session. As Dan Sullivan would say, "a win streak".

*3—**Improve my stay**—I know to put a blanket up on the window, cover the lights on the machines for night sleeping. I know to put a sign on the door with "patients name is Craig" not Richard (the R. in R. Craig Coppola). I know to put up a sign saying "nap in progress, please do not interrupt until ____", etc.*

*4—**change the vocabulary**. This is not a hospital stay, rather this is a "stay-cation". The chemo is not acid, rather it is my cancer fighting solders, etc.*

*5—**Plan for dinners**. I will have friends bring me dinners. Not just because the food is bad, but I need fellowship as well.*

Stay tuned to see if these work.

Write Your Own Algorithm on Your Care— Keep Writing It

Throughout my care, there were decision points that would change how my care was going to go. I strongly believe that you should start writing your own healthcare algorithm for each and every decision BEFORE you get to the juncture. If you are doing this, you can, without emotion, make rational decisions before they happen.

I remember going in for my third round of chemo, and the doctor wanted to adjust my dosage again to 177% of the initial dose. I thought that was fine, but then he said, "This will probably cause you to start getting blood transfusions." I had two minutes to decide. I HATED it. I should have been able to make that decision earlier and could have avoided the anxiety.

In the end, although I disliked the idea of transfusions, I trusted my doctor and we upped my dosage. But those are the kinds of decisions you'll be forced to make quickly, making it even more important that you have a team around you that you trust.

You have to get used to being in command of your care. Get comfortable and confident with making decisions on your terms, and no one else's.

Medical Resources

Tips for coping with cancer:
Mayo Clinic – www.mayoclinic.org

Newly diagnosed support:
Cancer Support Community
www.cancersupportcommunity.org

CaringBridge: www.caringbridge.org – Allows people to easily get updates on your journey and offer support and encouragement.

When someone you love is diagnosed with cancer:
http://www.rooshv.com/what-to-do-if-someone-close-to-you-gets-diagnosed-with-cancer

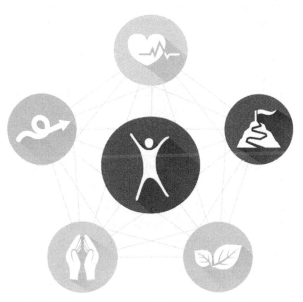

PRONG 2
SETTING GOALS

Set Goals—Big and Small

Cancer treatment is a time to set and reach goals. When you have some goals that are achievable during your treatment, it makes the treatment just another part of your day.

Having a goal to work towards gives your journey a positive arc. So many people spend their treatment lying around feeling sorry for themselves and only focusing on the negatives. But I can promise you that the more time you spend thinking about how sick you are, the sicker you will become.

Setting goals and working towards them allows you to put your mind to more productive and positive use. The time you spend in treatment will not feel wasted if you can accomplish even the smallest goal.

I set some big goals (publish two real estate books) and some small goals (reconnect with friends) and was happy I had the focus and drive to move them along during my chemo and other treatments. I promised myself that I would not look back at chemo and say I was not productive.

The goals I had during chemo were set before my first session and I modified them as I went through the process.

Below are examples of my goals. The first is a list of my big goals that I adjusted every week. Then, I included a list of specific goals I had for my second week in the hospital.

Big Goals:

1. Hike with no time limit. Hike early; get out in the dark because it's too hot to be in the sun. Start at 4–4:15. I can get two hours without much sun and catch a sunrise.

2. Have people to my house for lunch and a visit.

3. Write and catch up with people.

4. Deepen my connection with my kids.

5. Car camp.

6. Become an expert in meditation—download a number of healing tapes and meditation for my next hospital stay. My goal was to find the best and use them.

7. Change my diet for good.

8. Change my sleep habits and routine for good.

9. Create a new bucket list.

10. Be at peace.

Round two goals

1. Watch season two of *Game of Thrones.*

2. Get a minimum of two hours on the treadmill every day – but plan on three hours.

3. Give myself permission to watch as much TV and videos as I want.

4. Set up my hospital room the way I want (blanket in interior window, sign up for naps, sign up with my name, towels over machine lights).

5. Put meditation music on and meditate daily.

6. Use some weights and do body work. No pressure to do a lot, just to do it daily.

7. Have someone in for dinner every night.

8. Work on five small meals.

9. Sleep as much as I want. Finish stay with too much sleep rather than not enough.

Create Your Own Goals

I recommend creating your own goals for every stage of your treatment. Start with big picture goals you want to achieve in the long term. Then begin to break down those goals into smaller goals you can achieve during each round of treatment and during your off weeks between treatment.

I find that using the SMART goal outline is extremely helpful. SMART goals are:

Specific—Your goal should be worded very clearly, so there isn't any confusion about how to achieve it.

Measureable—Your goal should have a number attached to it. For example, lose 10 pounds or read three books. This makes it easier to track.

Attainable—For every goal you set, you need to also identify the steps you have to take to attain it. For example, if your goal is to read three books by the end of treatment, you have to break that down into smaller steps and commit to them. Reading ten pages a day, or a chapter each night, etc.

Realistic—This is a big one for goals set during cancer treatment. You have to pay attention to what your body says you can and can't do. For example, when I set the goal of lifting some weights, I gave myself room to go easy. I knew deadlifting 100 pounds wasn't attainable for me, so I set the bar a little lower to something I knew I could achieve.

Timely – Every goal should have a date attached to it. I set my goals by treatment weeks. I wanted to have a TV series watched by my last day in the hospital for that week. Without a deadline, you'll have little motivation to follow through on your goals.

There are many other online resources for creating goals, and countless books devoted to the topic. Take some time to define what you hope to accomplish over the next few weeks, and lay out a plan.

Reconnect with the Most Important People

One goal you absolutely can and should work towards during your treatment is reconnecting with the most important people in your life.

Take this time to reach out and connect with people who are important to you. They cannot say no. Take advantage of that. I organized 24 dinners at the hospital with my closest friends and team. Those two-hour dinners were great for me AND them. We each got to feel the love and connection of the relationship.

Not everyone has close family nearby or a large circle of friends, so remember that there are a lot of support groups and advocates available. This is *YOUR* plan. Find what works best for you, and make sure to surround yourself with people who will support you through it.

Generally, each hospital has patient advocates whose contact information can be found on the Patient Bill of Rights. These people are available to listen to and help you with your concerns, complaints, policies, and procedures, and to assist you in finding community services (moral support).

In addition to the resources at the hospital, The American Cancer Society® offers a number of services such as free rides to and from treatment and support groups that help when dealing with sensitive subjects or survivorship.

There are also outside groups that provide support with organized meetings for each individual type of cancer. These are offered in person at a set location outside of the hospital.

Life Doesn't Stop

Don't let your life stop because of your cancer. I've seen so many people who let their diagnosis steamroll them, and they spend months falling deeper and deeper into despair.

You have a choice about how you will spend your treatment. Will you let it dominate your life? Or will you take your life into your own hands?

Day Four, Round Two

Written August 22, 2013 4:48 p.m.

Thursday, August 22, 2013 –Day four of round two. I have one more overnight for this round and will be out by eight pm tomorrow. This staycation has been much smoother for me. My strategies are actually working. Ha. Planning for sure worked. Here are some highlights and a low light of the week:

A single low light—my hair. Gone. All of it. On day 17 of the first session it started falling out. Not uniform but clumps. The day before I checked in, I got the shears and took it down to a one. The closest to shaved as possible. I went one day in the hospital and was still losing it. I shaved it bald. Have to say, this was a bigger shock than I anticipated. Not because of hubris (ok, maybe a little) but more that this cancer and chemo is real. I am in the middle of the fight. I can tell you I have a TON more empathy for women. I was balding to begin with and I have had two days of pouting every time I look in the mirror.

I cannot imagine what it would be like to be female. I will forever give them all the credit. I vow to be over this and not look back by tomorrow at eight.

Highlights:

Since I shaved my head, I have been going outside (outside of the hospital) for 15 minutes of vitamin D for my scalp. I have a severely white head and need a little color before I am ready to face the world. I am calling it my daily jail break.

Meditation tapes. I have been meditating daily. I put a 45 minute CD on and found myself completely off mindfulness 4-5 times before the 30 minute mark. I have a ways to go, but heck I am trying.

So, one more night this trip. I feel good. More important (and as it turns out the most important check for the doctors) my blood counts have stayed good. Fingers crossed they stay that way.

Craig

PS—I do read and very much appreciate the guest entries. Many thanks for the thoughts, support and prayers.

Advocate/Support Group Resources:

Patient Advocate Groups: www.cscaz.org/
This is the Arizona website connected to Cancer Support Community, which is a local organization. Meetings are held on their campus. They do not provide in-hospital visits or support.

Rides to Treatment: www.cancer.org/
The American Cancer Society provides free rides with volunteer drivers to those who have no way to make it to treatments. You can find one close to you by searching your zip code at least four business days prior to your treatment.

They also offer information online about almost any question that could come up, including the sensitive subject of survivorship.

In-Hospital:

Generally, each hospital has patient advocates whose contact information can be found on the Patient Bill of Rights, which is provided by the hospital. These people are there to listen to you and help you with concerns, complaints, policies, procedures, and to assist you in finding community services (moral support). Via: www.hnfs.com/content/hnfs/home/tn/bene/res/patient_safety/patient_advocates.html

Family/Friend Support:

Lotsa Helping Hands: www.lotsahelpinghands.com/
This site allows you to create a care community. You can easily organize meals and help for friends and family in need. It provides coordination, communication, and support. This would be a great resource if your family or friends do not live nearby, so they can still be in your support group.

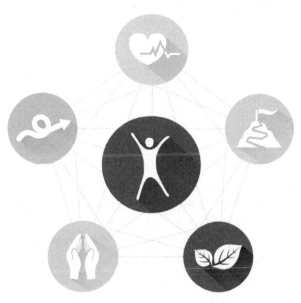

PRONG 3:
HOLISTIC APPROACH

Be Holistic

Cancer makes you feel all sorts of things. One of them is feeling like you are not in control. Taking control of what you can is a big part of getting your life back during and after treatments.

Being holistic means addressing all aspects of your mental, spiritual, emotional, and physical health. Often, in the journey to healing physically, we neglect the other parts of our lives that are just as important. That's why I made the effort to build in different kinds of treatments to my plan to make sure I was giving proper attention to all aspects of my health, and to "feel" like I had some semblance of control over the process.

Every alternative treatment I tried worked with my existing medical plan that I had put in place with my doctor. These treatments did not take the place of chemo, but instead allowed me to address other aspects of my health. Every decision I made was based upon how it fit into my plan. For example, I did not change my diet drastically during chemo because the doctors did not want me to lose weight. I did make some changes to be more conscious about what I was putting in my body, but for the most part did not take it to any extremes.

However, some people feel very strongly about adopting certain diets, whether that's vegetarian, vegan, or paleo, while they undergo treatment. It's about what works for you and your plan.

I received a lot of homeopathic doctor referrals from all sorts of people who swore by them. In the end, I did not go with anybody, but preferred to put together my own holistic plan (along with the integrative medicine doctor at MD Anderson), picking and choosing alternative treatments that I felt helped me.

If you want to consult a homeopathic doctor, there are plenty of options out there. The key is to make sure all the members of your team are working together for YOU. Make sure to consult your primary medical doctor before you commit to or try any homeopathic options.

Below I go through a few of the holistic treatments that I explored. You may be interested in some and not others, or want to go looking for more. Find what works for you.

Acupuncture

Acupuncture is one widely-touted treatment that can help with the side effects of treatment. It has been known to help with pain control and the extreme nausea that occurs during chemo. It can increase blood flow and reduce swelling and aid constipation.

I did acupuncture both in and out of the hospital. There was an acupuncturist employed by the hospital where I did treatment, and I got to know her well during my stays.

While this is a physical activity, I turned it in to a mind/ spirit exercise. I'm not sure how effective it was but I believe I was more relaxed and had a better outlook when I was done.

Of course the effects will be different for everyone, so you might start by consulting an acupuncturist who is trained to treat cancer patients. And as with all additional treatments, make sure you run it by your doctor first. You never know how your treatment plan might make you react to different stimuli.

Massage

Chemo can induce anxiety and tension (in addition to a ton of other maladies), which manifests in your body in different ways. Massage is one way you can release that tension and relax.

Like acupuncture, massage has also been shown to help with pain, nausea, and fatigue. All of which are side effects of cancer treatment. Massage can also help alleviate some of the emotional side effects of a cancer diagnosis, such as anxiety, fear, and depression, by helping you relax and let go.

Because I had lymphoma, a cancer that affects your lymphatic system, I frequently did lymphatic massages, which drain your lymph nodes and reduce swelling.

If your treatment is causing you anxiety or pain, consult your doctor to see if massage might help you reduce tension.

Homeopathy

Homeopathy refers to consuming different substances from nature to heal certain physical traits.

Many cancer patients swear by homeopathy, and believe that certain herbs have tremendous benefits to combatting the side effects of treatment.

If you are interested in homeopathy, consult an expert. Don't try to do it yourself by Googling herbs and then going to your local farmer's market and testing them out.

Cancer treatment is complex, and everyone's treatment will be different. Some substances could have negative effects when paired with certain medicines, so make sure you consult with your primary cancer doctor at every turn.

There have been tremendous successes in treating symptoms with homeopathy, but remember to only do what works for you and your treatment.

Diet

I avoided homeopathy, but I did make conscious decisions about what I put in my body.

I interviewed two naturopathic doctors and selected one. I had two former doctors that turned to the natural path, and MD Anderson, the hospital where I received my treatment, had its own integrative medicine headed by Dr. Diljeet Singh.

I started by taking Vitamin D, and still take it on my doctor's advice. Vitamin D is a big marker in lymphoma, and mine was really low. Getting outside daily was also recommended to help me increase my Vitamin D intake.

While I avoided major dietary changes, I still was put on two low-maintenance diets during the treatments. First they put me on a low microbial diet during chemo. I didn't have white blood cells to fight any foreign objects, so I needed some help. This diet excluded any salads or fruit that were not double hand washed, meat had to be cooked to at least 165 degrees, and nothing fresh could be eaten at restaurants.

Then, I went on a low fiber diet for radiation. Because the mass was in my abdomen, I could not afford to have a big stomach, gas or a lot of water in my system. I scheduled the earliest times I could and ate my latest meal before 7 pm. The biggest concerns were: overeating and coming in with a big stomach, drinking too much water, eating too much cabbage, beans (can you believe), peanut butter, whole grains, bran, raw vegetables and most nuts.

I received no less than 20 emails from well-wishers sending along the miracle food to eat that would cure cancer or prevent cancer. Yes, turmeric is good to put in your cooking. And broccoli is great. Grass fed beef is the preferred beef, etc. But the doctors and nutritionists that I met with were pretty adamant—there is no miracle food. So with that premise, here are some tips from the dieticians from Banner MD Anderson and MD Anderson. Most, if not all, you have probably seen before.

- Stay on the outside aisles of the store—the closer the food is to the ground the better; all those foods are on the outside aisles.

- If you buy processed foods, compare ingredients and choose the food with: the shortest ingredient list, ingredients you can pronounce, and the least amount of added sugar, fat and salt.

- Choose whole foods where possible.

- Eating healthy takes time (time to shop, and cook). Plan ahead.

- They seem to like a plant based diet (which includes beans, nuts and whole grains), men 7-11 servings a day and women 5-8.

- 3/4 of your plate to be filled with the plant items –rainbow color your veggies.

- Limit red meat to 2 times (18 oz.) a week.

- Fish, poultry or beans are a great alternative source of protein.

Meditation and Breathing

Stress can counteract all of your traditional and non-traditional treatments, so including practices that help reduce stress is always a good idea. Meditation and yoga are two activities you can include in your daily routine.

I prayed, meditated, visualized, and focused on my healing. All of these helped me move along the healing path.

Lots of people want to know about meditation. Many find it very difficult to find the time or patience to commit to meditation, but it doesn't have to be difficult. In the book Praying Naked, the first chapter is about 3-minute meditation in the shower. Sometimes, all it takes is a few minutes to center yourself and let go of anxiety.

If you want the seminal book on meditation (granted the name is atrocious) check out *Full Catastrophe Living* by Jon Kabat-Zinn. This is the best, most down-to-earth and easy process for meditation. I really connected with it, and still follow it for daily meditation.

An important part of taking control of your life during and after treatments is working on your belief system or your mind. Stay in the moment. This means not focusing on what happened yesterday or what could happen tomorrow. As Louise Hay says, "Your power is in the present moment."

This leads me to using positive affirmations during all treatments. If you believe that your treatments are doing their job and helping your healing process, then they will. Some examples are:

- My body is returning to its natural state of health.

- My healing treatments are restoring my body to a healthy state.

- Every day and in every way, I am getting healthier and healthier.

I also spent almost every day working on my breathing and trying to either meditate, become connected, be present, or get through a tough period. I cannot say enough about the immediate and cumulative effects of taking mindful breaths throughout the day and especially during rough patches.

Yoga

There are so many different kinds of Yoga for every mood/capability. Do a little research and find one that works for you during this time.

I had practiced yoga for years before my diagnosis. During treatment I decided to do yoga that was less active and more restorative. It became less about the workout and more about my mind-body connection.

Yoga is a great way to deepen your connection with your body. Plus, if you have trouble meditating on your own, Yoga instructors can help guide you through basic meditation to help you clear your mind.

Physical Activity

Movement is also a key component to a holistic lifestyle.

- Be active. Keep moving. Walking or hiking is one activity you can easily work into your schedule and you don't need any special equipment to do it.

- As I've said before, I hit the trail every time I left the hospital. This not only got me moving, but it helped me reclaim my life after spending a week as a patient.

- I also tried to workout in the hospital, hitting the treadmill for as long as my doctor felt comfortable. Again, I included my doctor in my workout plans to make sure I didn't overdo it.

Before treatment, I was extremely active, and the biggest challenge for me was to let go when I could not do what I wanted to. I thought for sure I would be jogging, yoga, weight lifting during my treatment, but I had to let go of some of those expectations and be happy with what I could do.

So stay active and moving, but give yourself grace when those things are hard.

Social

When you're battling cancer, your world naturally becomes narrower. It is limited to doctors, nurses, the hospital, family, and a select group of friends, and sometimes not even that. Sometimes you go days without talking to people other than doctors and nurses.

Cancer is lonely.

To counter this feeling, I planned dinners in the hospital, one-on-one meetings at my home office, and regular phone calls with friends and family. I am not normally a person who needs constant companionship, but being thrown off my normal routine was hard, and I had to work to incorporate those regular social connections into my schedule.

You can't neglect your social self. It's another area that you have to address in your holistic approach. When I couldn't see friends and family, I attended classes at MD Anderson like Laughter for Health, Nutrition for Individuals Affected by Cancer, and Tibetan Bon

Meditation. Being around other people helped me feel less alone, and made a big difference in the long run.

Other Ideas

Imagine your treatment as your own personal band of warriors. Chemo became my cancer warrior and Rituxan became my personal Navy Seals team. Changing my mindset about small things like this helped me face each round of chemo with a little more confidence.

While your treatment is hard at work attacking your cancer, you can find time to build in a little relaxation into your schedule.

You can also think of your time in the hospital for treatments as a staycation and use it to relax, recharge, and be positive. You might binge watch a new television show, have a spa day, or take this time to read a new book.

Know that where you are in your journey is the perfect place. Your healing is going at just the right speed.

I began to tackle each day at "Tashi pace." Tashi was my head Sherpa when I trekked to the Mount Everest Base Camp. I wanted to hike faster and told him so.

Tashi replied, "This pace is fine."

Let this pace be fine.

Holistic is not a term that just describes your treatment but your entire lifestyle. Your body needs plenty of rest to heal. Strive to get at least seven hours of sleep each night and nap daily.

Make your journey a mindful one. Remain mindful every day, hour, and with every breath. Remember, do not look back or forward but to the now.

Resource:

A Survivor's Guide to Kicking Cancer's Ass by Dena Mendes

Update/ Holistic Approach

Written January 25, 2014 10:38 a.m.

Today is on a topic that everybody seems to have an opinion, a solution, or a story to tell. How to fight cancer with an integrative approach not just medicine. I have been trying to take a Holistic approach to fighting cancer. Here is what I have learned—There seems to be three major areas where integrative medicine is focused:

Physical—this includes the biggest areas of diet, physical activity, etc.

Mind-Spirit—This includes meditation, music, breathing, and praying.

Social—What you do and who you do it with. Cancer patients lives can get very narrow during and after treatment.

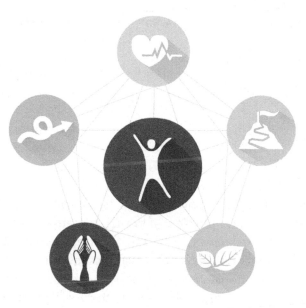

PRONG 4: SPIRITUAL CONSIDERATIONS

Begin to Pray and Seek Love

During the treatment and the entire cancer ordeal, I found you start to question a lot of things. The world that once seemed so secure and dependable is thrown into chaos, and every day brings uncertainties. How will you feel today? Is your treatment working? How is your blood count? Will you feel well enough to see your friends?

You're going to face a lot of uncertainties, which is why it's so important to have a constant in your life that goes beyond earthly understanding. Something powerful that remains steady when everything else becomes turbulent.

Spirituality is a personal path we all take. No matter your beliefs or religious inclinations, we all have a spiritual life that we must define and build for ourselves.

Deepening your spirituality has tremendous benefits emotionally and physically. In fact, a meta-analysis of 42 studies examining over 125,000 people published by the American Psychological Association in 2000, found that attendance at a place of worship, any place of worship, can add eight years to the average life span AND significantly improve health. Prayer has also been found to lower breathing and heart rates and reduce blood pressure.

In his really cool book, *Deep Survival: Who Lives, Who Dies, and Why*, Laurence Gonzales talks to survivors of all kinds of challenges. Faith is a very important factor in people's will to survive. "Whether a deity is actually listening or not, there is value in formally announcing your needs, desires, worries, sins, and goals in a focused prayerful attitude."

But how we reach that spiritual level is a different path for everyone. Maybe you cultivate your spiritual self through organized religion, or by deepening your personal relationship with God. Maybe it's by experiencing a deeper connection to nature and the greater cosmos. Spirituality may also take shape in the relationships you have with other people.

However you define spirituality in your life, it will become an important cornerstone during your cancer treatment.

Discovering My Spiritual Path

I am a Christian, so for me, this process was about growing my understanding of God and Jesus Christ, and how I could define Him in my personal life. How could I connect more to Him? How could I be at peace with the process?

I started reading a lot about prayer, meditation, and spirituality. The more I read, the more I found my path.

Meditation

During my treatment I was open to practices from other religions and spiritual paths that I could bring into my own understanding of God. For example, I practiced meditation to put my mind at ease and to help cope with the rigorous treatments. This became a spiritual act for me, and helped me calm my soul.

Bruce Feller, in his book *Abraham*, talks to Christian theologian Walter Brueggemann who says (I paraphrase): It is perfectly legitimate for Christians to draw all traditions to Jesus, no matter their origin. So Buddhist meditation can be used to further Christianity.

Like everything else in my treatment, I had to find practices that worked for me, to help me define myself as a spiritual person and reach a deeper level of connectivity with my faith.

I received recommendations from those I knew who practiced mediation. I downloaded a variety of meditation resources, and then put it in my plan to meditate at least three times a week.

This practice was strengthened when I was reading Paramhansa Yogananda in his book *Autobiography of a Yogi*.

Throughout almost the entire book he takes time to share the parallels of Buddhism and Christianity. On the eve of his first trip to the U.S., his master says to him, "Forget you were born a Hindu, and don't be an American. Take the best of them both. Be your true self, a child of God. Seek and incorporate into your being the best qualities of all your brothers scattered over the earth in various races."

Bringing meditation into my spiritual practice helped me to center myself and live in the current moment, instead of living in fear of the next moment.

They asked the Buddha to sum up enlightenment in one word. He replied: "Awareness." Asked to elaborate, he replied: "Awareness is awareness is awareness."

Wake up. Be aware. Be present. Sounds a lot like meditation to me.

Prayer

I also spent time strengthening my ability to pray, at all times of the day, asking for help when I needed it and giving thanks for every breath.

I pulled out a book I have owned for over a decade and never read. The book drove everything home for me. It was so good, I have ordered a number to give to those who have been helping me along my spiritual journey. The book is from the teachings of an Indian-born Jesuit priest Anthony De Mello. De Mello passed away in 1987 but his words and work live on. It's called *Praying Naked* by J. Francis Stroud, S.J.

The teachings are simple, direct, and hit me right between the eyes. Stroud says almost all exercises are to get the "pray-er" or meditator into the present. In a sense that is what all teachers of prayer try to do –to get you to live in the present where God is.

He is neither in the past nor in the future, neither of which exist, but in the present. So if you can get into the present, you can easily get in touch with God.

Thomas Carlyle said, "The tragedy of life is not how much we suffer. But how much we miss!" By honing my ability to pray and live in gratitude in each moment, I not only found a deeper connection to God, but I was able to achieve a level of peace I didn't think would be possible during cancer treatment.

Nature

As I've said before, I am a long distance backpacker. One of my goals every year, and during my treatment, was to sleep on the ground, and to catch as many sunrises as I could.

Backpacking becomes a spiritual experience for me. Sleeping outside, surrounded by nature and underneath a sky full of brilliant stars helps me establish a sense of peace. The world can be so chaotic, that disconnecting and getting off the grid becomes important particularly during times of extreme stress.

At the end of each of my hospital stays, I headed straight for the trails to reclaim my life and find that deeper sense of calm and connection.

Remember that you are in charge of your life. Find your peace, your space, and your spirit. However you define spirituality, practice it daily.

Spiritual Resources:

Books:

- *Praying Naked* by Anthony De Mello
- The Untethered Soul: The Journey Beyond Itself by Michael A. Singer
- The Autobiography of a Yogi by Paramahansa Yoganand

Meditation Resources:

Books:

- Success Through Stillness by Russell Simmons
- *Thrive* by Arianna Huffington
- The Miracle of Mindfulness: An Introduction to the Practice of Meditation by Thich Nhat Hanh

Audio:

- Guided Mindfulness Meditation
  (www.mindfulnesscds.com)

- *Silva UltraMind* (www.silvaultramind.com)

- *Eckhart Tolle* (www.eckharttolle.com)

- *Headspace* app (for meditation)
  (www.headspace.com)

Video:

- De Mello videos www.demellospirituality.com

- There is a fantastic interview by Oprah with Thich
  Nhat Hanh, a Vietnamese Buddhist monk on
  Youtube if you search "Oprah Winfrey talks with
  Thich Nhat Hanh Excerpt   Powerful"

Spiritual Thoughts / Update

Written January 3, 2014 4:30 p.m.

When I was diagnosed with lymphoma in late July, I had a four prong approach to beating cancer: 1— medically, 2—homeopathic changes in my life, 3— lifestyle changes, and 4—spiritually. This post is my attempt (albeit clumsy I know) to put these past six months into words from my spiritual focus. I loved this quote from Paul Salopek who is on a seven year journey by foot to trace human migration: "I am on a journey. I am in pursuit of an idea, a story, a chimera....." I too want this to be a journey.

First a few points of reference:

1. I am a Christian.

2. I have always been interested in other religions, not to change mine, but I like aspects of other religions and had been incorporating them into my life before the diagnosis.

3. I am completely open to all prayers, religions and spirituality from everyone I know. I want the group strength added to mine. And I believe in all prayer to anybody's God.

I have been truly amazed by the breadth and depth of the prayers I've received from all religions. It has been powerful....

My chimera: How can I deepen my faith, use it to strengthen my resolve to fight my lymphoma, and finally to reconcile my life long desire to take the best of all religions and use them to my benefit. Sound simple? Actually, it has been.

Banner Gateway Hospital sends chaplains by twice a week. Chaplain Joe, a small unassuming Italian and I hit it off. I think it would be fair to say Joe hits it off with everybody. Every conversation was intimate and interesting.

Joe said the one thing he did not like about religion was the "religiosity." He said that to him, he just wanted to talk to God. Put everything else aside. Just talk to Him. I like that. I had connected with Jesus Today, the daily reader and Jesus Calling, the iPhone app by Sarah Young. Simple.

The journey continues....

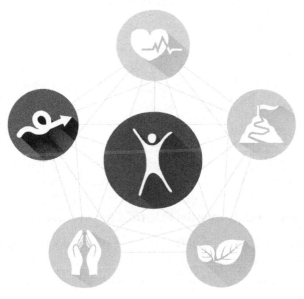

PRONG 5:
EXPECT THE UNEXPECTED

Murphy's Law

This prong is the Murphy's Law Prong; things that came up that I could not plan for. These were all things that I did not think about at the beginning, but were very important at the end.

The most unexpected part of your cancer diagnosis is the actual diagnosis. No one expects to hear they have cancer, which is why throughout this entire book I've advocated creating a plan right away so you can get a firm handle on it.

You will find your own method of getting through treatment. You will find mantras, practices, relationships, faiths, and more that will help you conquer this process. You will also encounter unique obstacles and hurdles that you will have to overcome.

This prong includes a few unexpected areas in my life that I didn't consider before treatment, as well as some tips that helped me navigate the process as a whole.

Communicating with Friends and Family

Handling your family in this type of situation is, in my opinion, the hardest part. How do you keep others updated on your health without creating a huge chore for yourself?

I didn't realize how time consuming this part of the treatment would be. Everyone wants to know how you're doing, how they can help, and what you need. What do you tell them? How do you balance the precious time you have to yourself with making sure the people you love are ok?

Set your communication guidelines from the start, and keep them consistent throughout the entire process. For my immediate family, I chose the "You Know What I Know" method, keeping them up to date after every appointment.

There were no secrets in my treatment, and still, in remission, I continue to keep them updated after every scan and appointment. Some of the hardest calls were to my kids right after bad news. The kids wanted to know that I was not pulling any punches or keeping things from them. They wanted to be informed. To tell my children was a conscious decision that I made at the beginning of the process, and it worked well for me.

This was very hard during the bad-news calls and meetings and a whole lot easier during the good-news calls and meetings. I believe it created trust and they knew I would leave nothing out, therefore there would be no sudden surprises—good or bad.

This method got a bit trickier when extended family and friends started reaching out. While I wanted to keep them informed, I also didn't have the time or stamina to individually communicate updates to each person. Which leads me to my next point.

Guard Your Lucid Time for Priorities

Not surprisingly, people want your time—nurses in the hospital, doctors on rounds, the chaplain, the therapy dog, the oncologist, the PA—and that is just during the hospital stay. Friends, family (not immediate), and well-wishers can all take time, and you only have a little time each day to be present. Live your priorities by spending your lucid time on those items.

In the middle of my chemo, I sat down with my youngest daughter, Claire, and told her what my priorities were in order. They were: me and my health, Mom (so she could help me and the family), and then Claire. It wasn't her brother and sisters, but her. Why? She was the only kid still at home; I needed to be involved with her. I had little to no time left over for anything or anybody else.

That didn't mean I didn't care about other friends and family, or want to keep them informed on my treatment as well. I just didn't have the time or capacity to keep every single person in my life in the know.

One way I found to keep my friends and extended family updated was to set up a CaringBridge account (www.caringbridge.org). This is a free website that is essentially a blog, so your family, friends, colleagues, and neighbors can follow your journey. Everyone who cares and wants to know how you are doing can follow you and stay up-to-date on your progress.

Yes, it takes time and dedication to write the posts, and sometimes (a lot of the time) I didn't feel up to it. But my motivation was reading all of the responses and well wishes I received after I sent out an update. This reassured me that everyone was pulling for me. It helped us feel connected, even if we weren't talking directly.

Written July 28, 2013

Communications: for now, I am trying to focus on getting the correct diagnosis and starting the treatment. I also spent last week turning over the businesses to my team. That is my main focus. Once I get going on the chemo, I am sure I will have more time. For now, please limit the well wishes to texts and emails to Tracy until I get into treatment later this week. I have found myself losing sight of what needs to be done. Today is the 14th day after I noticed a lump on my neck. I have been racing to get everything taken care of. I want to make sure I am focused on getting completely committed to the healing process.

Give Yourself Grace—Lots of It

"Accept where you are. Use what you have. Do what you can." I was given this quote from a friend and found it extremely useful.

You will not feel great all the time. When you do not feel great, let it go. I found myself getting a lot done during the early rounds of chemo. As the cumulative effect took hold, I just gave myself more and more grace. Emails stacked up, my weekly marketing articles went unwritten, and I stayed on the treadmill less and less. But you know what? I was okay with not getting anything done.

Breathe and find your peace. Peace is the place where you know you have done what you can, figured out what you need to do, you get on the path, and then you let it go.

A friend of mine learned this lesson first hand when he began his cancer journey. His process included a lot of growth, and he shared some hard truths that he faced with me:

1. You can't be yourself right now. You can't be the dad you want, the husband, employee, son or son in law, that you want to be.

2. You can't help like you used to. Whatever your role in your family used to be, whether as the man in the house or caretaker, you can't do it right now.

3. Some days, you can't hit even small goals. Give yourself some grace.

Once he came to terms with these realizations, he learned some great lessons:

1. You can and will get through this.

2. You have to give yourself grace to not be you right now.

3. You can learn to be other things. An inspiration, a loving and kind friend, etc.

4. You can grow during this time.

And yes, you learn self-depreciating humor.

See Reality as It Is, and Plan Accordingly

Some people close to me wanted to think everything would be okay, but that is not always the case. You are in charge of your health. You have to see reality, and you have to make the tough decisions. If you start the process of seeing reality early on, then you can continue throughout. You have to make the ultimate decision; do it with reality in mind.

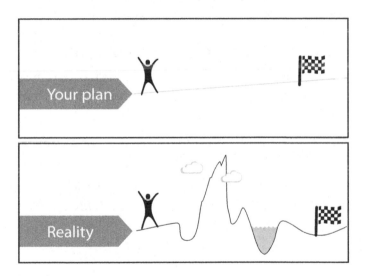

Without seeing reality, you aren't able to plan. And as I've said time and time again, you need a plan. Plan for everything, not just remission. It's not pleasant and it's not easy, but you have to be prepared for every outcome.

Tree-to-Tree Running

When the going gets tough, do what ultra-runners do: Run tree-to-tree. Just commit to getting to the next milestone, and then reset for another milestone.

You have to keep looking forward in small increments. If you're constantly looking at the big picture, it's easy to get overwhelmed by doubt and anxiety. So just focus on the next step, getting through the next treatment or even just this moment. You can make it.

The Nadir Will Happen Again and Again

You will hit bottom, and then there will be another bottom lower than the last. This will continue. Accept it.

na·dir: (nādər,nādir/) noun

The lowest point in the fortunes of a person or organization."they had reached the nadir of their sufferings"

Cumulative Is a Bitch—Plan for It

Treatment is designed to take you to your knees. When you buckle, recognize where you are, and then pray. It will happen. And when it does, it will most likely take you by surprise.

Like everything else, have a plan for this moment. Find your strength and store it up for when you need it. That's why I recommend trying different things early, while you're still feeling good, so that when the worst happens you know what works to lift you back up.

Dodging Bullets

Written October 14, 2013 4:58 p.m.

Round four chemo (plus IV) continues to kick butt, mine and I am positive the cancer cells as well. I am positive because I am sitting here on Monday afternoon 11 days after I got out of the hospital and I am still nauseous. The chemo HAS to be working. My white blood count was at .2 last week. I figure there was a week where I had to be cancer free. No white cells, good or bad, no cancer.

The doctors warned me this round would be the first round that most likely would require blood or platelet transfusions. Well, Friday, my counts were good enough to not get one AND this morning they were again. Dodged two bullets in the past 72 hours. How did I do it? Simple plan….Shut it down. I have been sleeping 18-20 hours a day. Letting my body recover.

Listen to Your Words— They Tell You Where You Are

What you tell your friends, family, and doctors is where you are. Listen to yourself as you talk. You will know.

Yes It's a Roller Coaster—Ride It, Then Get Off; Ride It, Then Get Off

I really dislike roller coasters. I hate the drops and turns, but knowing that I can see the track ahead, and prepare for when those high points and low points are coming, makes a huge difference. It's the same with your cancer treatment. If you can look ahead and prepare for the highs and lows, and the times when you get off, you control the ride.

Normalize the process as much as possible. When you are on chemo, ride it. When the chemo is done, get off, and get back to your life and to yourself.

I want to emphasize the last part—you have to get off the roller coaster. You can't keep riding it during your off weeks. You have to reclaim your life between treatments, otherwise you'll just keep going in circles.

Transition

Written December 4, 2013 5:15 p.m.

This weekend, I started the transition from knee buckling treatments to getting my life back. Yes, I know I have 22 radiation treatments to do. Yes, I know I have to move to Houston for the month of January. But, why not get started now? I had a chuckle to myself as I typed that. I always start my annual business and personal plan on or before Halloween and have it completed for the following year before Thanksgiving. Why would this be any different?

I want to transition my life, not necessarily back to where it was, but to where I want/need it to be. AND I want to transition this CaringBridge to make sure I am not dragging it out or cutting off from what the people I most care about want to know.

I am sure more to follow on my life in the future but, this topic is the difficult one. I have a crazy successful business now beginning my 30th year. But, that business is very consuming and stressful. I will be working on these areas over the next couple months as I heal.

For the journal entries, I thought I would commit to updating my story on a weekly basis—no more. I sincerely hope there is very little to update on me personally. During these weekly updates, I will add a second part. Some part of this process that has been meaningful to me. Topics include some education I have received on cancer, chemo, stem cells or radiation. I might also have some additional thoughts on caregiving, physical appearance, mental acuity during chemo, or mental states of chemo brain.

The personal update will be the first item and if you are busy you can skip the rest. So, over the next two months until I get the sign I am done, you can stay engaged and maybe I can help some of you as you sadly but inevitably have to deal with cancer in your life—your own or a close relative/friend.

Thanks for the continued support and the guestbook updates. I read each and every one of them with our friendship in mind.

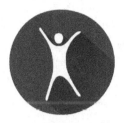

After Surviving Cancer

It's been over three years now, and I'm happy to say that I'm doing great. However, my cancer is a 10-year watch and hope. It's always in the back of my mind.

I was asked recently if there is anything I would do differently if I had to do it over again. I can honestly say I am very pleased with the plan I put together. I'm happy with the priorities I set for myself, and the way I handled treatment. While you are fighting this battle, there are all sorts of mental, emotional, and physical changes happening in your life. It can be easy to just sort of give in and let 'the system' take over.

But this is your journey, and you get to do it the way you want to do it. This book isn't for me, or for anybody, to say, "This how you need to do it." Rather, think of this book as permission for you to get organized, despite the emotion that comes along with a cancer diagnosis. This is your process, your direction, and ultimately, your life. Empower yourself to go down that path.

All these lessons still apply after surviving cancer. God willing, if you make it through the process to the other side, you have to take back your life and live it the way you want to. If and when you receive that second chance, make the most of it.

Your Post-Cancer Plan

Taking back your life after surviving cancer requires a plan just as detailed as your plan for treatment. It means looking ahead, preparing for scans and appointments, but also making sure you live your life the way you want it.

After receiving that last, clean scan that marked the end of my cancer treatment, I established a plan that was just a thorough as my cancer plan. It included the following steps:

1. **Get my health back.** Recovering from the toxicity of the chemo and the radiation took time. My white blood counts were still low, my strength and stamina sucked, and my weight was too high. I still needed naps several days a week. Recovering from treatment was a process that took a while, and remained my top priority.

2. **Eat Healthy.** Enough said.

3. **Move forward.** Cancer has yet to define me. I will not let it. Period. Sherri Magee and Kathy Scalzo say it well in their book, *Picking Up the Pieces, Moving Forward After Surviving Cancer*: "Recovery is not so much about moving on as it is about moving through

change.....Recovery phase is centered on healing the person."

4. **Find my New Normal.** I became focused and looked forward to the next stage in my life. It was a new opportunity to, once again, redefine myself.

"Many survivors feel incredible pressure from within, as well as from others, to return to their old self, to 'get back to being the person we know and Love.' Family and friends are as surprised and unprepared as you are for the lingering side effects of fatigue, sadness or confusion. All they want is to breathe a sigh of relief, celebrate your victory over cancer, and move on. Unfortunately, this isn't going to happen.... For many survivors, the redefinition of identity is a process that moves through several stages. You will need time to adapt to each new phase." (Sherri Magee and Kathy Scalz)

5. **Learn to live with uncertainty.** I spent the first six weeks after treatment looking over my shoulder. Eventually, I had to stop.

"During treatment, most survivors simply live from one day to the next. But part of recovery—resuming everyday life—necessarily involves looking ahead... They wish everything could go back to the way it used to be... They long for the innocence and security they see as coming from not having to face your own mortality—even if that innocence and security are false." (Sherri Magee and Kathy Scalz)

De-bunking two myths

There are two myths about life after cancer that I wish to de-bunk here:

"Cancer rules your life"

You will never truly get away from your cancer, even if you go into remission for the rest of your life. There will be scans, yearly check-ins, and every time you fill out your medical history it will be flagged. But cancer does not rule your life.

Deal with your anxiety, book your doctors' appointments and scans, and then move forward. Don't let your cancer control your life. Reclaim your life for yourself.

"Cancer defines you"

You don't have to be known as "the cancer guy." You define yourself. This is another reason I set goals for myself during my treatment that had nothing to do with my medical diagnosis. I wanted to accomplish things that defined me as a person, not a patient or a victim.

It bears repeating: You define yourself. You write your own story. Make it a good one.

After-Treatment Books:

Picking Up the Pieces: Moving Forward After Surviving Cancer by Sherri Magee, PH. D and Kathy Scalzo, M.S. O.D.

A Survivor's Guide to Kicking Cancer's Ass by Dena Mendes

The Cancer Survivor's Companion: Practical Ways to Cope with Your Feelings After Cancer by Lucy Atkins and Francis Goodhart

Written March 21, 2014 2:18 p.m.

Great news!! I was in Houston yesterday for my PET scan six weeks after finishing radiation. For the first time, I received a negative PET Scan indicating I am Cancer free. Feels good to type that. Cancer free!!! In no way do I want to be a buzz kill from the good news. I am excited, relieved, grateful, humbled, and happy all at the same time. That said, I have to learn to live with the fact that I have some decent odds of facing cancer again. I know time is the best healer of this and acknowledge I need time to fully incorporate all the thoughts and feelings into my life. I have Lymphoma. The oncologists believe I had Large cell B (curable) and have follicular (not curable). I have been to hell and back getting 720 hours of chemo drip and 22 sessions of radiation—All of it necessary to get me to this place—Cancer free. Now the task is to stay cancer free. The doctors believe the odds are 65-80 percent I will get long term (five year or more) remission. If I can stay in remission for a long time, there is a good chance of new drugs, new procedures, or even a cure. I am now going into post cancer mode. I have spent quite a bit of time working on this over the past two months.

Actually, I am pretty excited. I constantly tell my kids to be comfortable with being uncomfortable.

The past six weeks have been very interesting in terms of trying to become more mindful and less future driven. I must have breathed in March 21st, and let it go over 1,000 times. When I got into this cancer treatment process, I thought I was at least the equivalent of a freshman in high school at meditation and being mindful. As it turns out, I was, maybe a 5th or 6th grader. "We believe a simple, consistent daily practice that integrates body, mind, heart and spirit is an essential first step to recovering a sense of wholeness." I am now very focused on this for my next steps/priorities.

A Final Word

Cancer is a chapter in your life. Just a chapter. There are many chapters as you move through the process. Be sure to keep looking forward, and as my coach says, "Make your future bigger than your past."

If you enjoyed this book

please share your opinion

with others on Amazon.com.

We would love to hear

what you have to say

and greatly appreciate

your support.

Made in the USA
Coppell, TX
08 March 2020